The Ultimate Strength Training Nutrition Guide: This Will Take You To The Next Level

Introduction

I want to thank you and congratulate you for downloading the book, *Training Nutrition Guide that will take you to the Next Level.*

This book contains proven steps and strategies on how to go on a proper diet that is required by your body to get the best out of workout.

This book also contains a list of some healthy and very important food you're your body requires especially if you work out regularly. This book also provides information about the perfect timing to eat what to eat to get the best out of your training.

Thanks again for downloading this book, I hope you enjoy it!

© Copyright 2019 by Stephen Jones All rights reserved.

This document is geared towards providing reliable information based on studies and research in regards to the topic and issue covered. Any information or advice given within this book may change overtime. The author will not be held reliable for any action or results that the reader may decide to take upon the given information. The publication is sold with the idea that the publisher is not required to render accounting, officially permitted, or otherwise, qualified services. If advice is necessary, legal or professional, a practiced individual in the profession should be ordered.

- From a Declaration of Principles which was accepted and approved equally by a Committee of the American Bar Association and a Committee of Publishers and Associations.

In no way is it legal to reproduce, duplicate, or transmit any part of this document in either electronic means or in printed format. Recording of this publication is strictly prohibited and any storage of this document is not allowed unless with written permission from the publisher. All rights reserved.

The information provided herein is stated to be truthful and consistent, in that any liability, in terms of inattention or otherwise, by any usage or abuse of any policies, processes, or directions contained within is the solitary and utter responsibility of the recipient reader. Under no circumstances will any legal responsibility or blame be held against the publisher for any reparation, damages, or monetary loss due to the information herein, either directly or indirectly.

Respective authors own all copyrights not held by the publisher.

The information herein is offered for informational purposes solely, and is universal as so. The presentation of the information is without contract or any type of guarantee assurance.

The trademarks that are used are without any consent, and the publication of the trademark is without permission or backing by the trademark owner. All trademarks and brands within this book are for clarifying purposes only and are the owned by the owners themselves, not affiliated with this document.

Chapter 1 (Nutrients Requirement)

Insert Workout done every day is a great way to stay healthy. It keeps your body fit and smart, it also adds to your beauty, awesome right! When talking about nutrition, considering the different hypothesis about nutrients requirement out there, knowing what fact is and what is fiction can be really confusing. But in this book, I'd be stating facts that have been tested and confirmed to work. Although, giving a nutritional guide to a vast amount of individual might not really be exerting but trial and error to figure out what's optimal. Also, giving a nutritional guide to just an individual that you know personally makes the whole process easier cause a nutritional guide can be given to a person on the bases of the person calories intake, the rate at which the body uses calories, the actions of the person, immunity etc. Generally, how we handle and use nutrient is the key in figuring out what nutritional guide works best for you.

Nutrition is not a topic that can be wrapped up in just one topic or one book, nutrition is vast and broad. So you need to read broad, wide and keep yourself updated with ongoing research. For example, an article might talk about the nutritional requirement for a 20-year-old male body builder weighing 250lb hoping to improve his body physique, which when compared with a 40-year old woman training for a marathon, they both require different nutrient in what they eat. Some people might just simply reduce the number of carbohydrates they consume and it helps them greatly, others might increase their carbohydrates consumption and still flourish. For some, it is when the fat in their food is reduced. Many individuals have also confirmed that when they eat frequently say every 2-3 hours, it works just as well for them.

Our body consists of lots of muscles. Every movement made, no matter how small is as a result of a muscle contracting or expanding. For a muscle to contract, energy must be involved and it is derived from glucose in the form of a substance called Adenosine Triphosphate (ATP). Adenosine Trisphosphate (ATP) is gotten from the food we eat.

When oxygen is used in the catabolism of Adenosine Triphosphate to produce energy, water and carbon dioxide are produced as the by-products. These by-products can be excreted from the body either through the skin, lung or kidney, or it could be reused by the body wherever needed. The process whereby the muscles use oxygen to break down Adenosine Triphosphate which produces energy is called aerobic energy production.

When the body cannot produce the required oxygen needed for the catabolism of Adenosine Triphosphate to produce energy, it switches into a different system of producing energy where oxygen is not needed in the catabolism of Adenosine Triphosphate. When oxygen is not used to break down Adenosine Triphosphate, a different product called lactic acid is produced as a by-product. The lactic acid is responsible for the aches we feel in our muscles after vigorous activity. The process whereby the muscles do not use oxygen to break down Adenosine Triphosphate to produce energy is called anaerobic energy production.

When we are carrying out our normal daily routine, the body can make use of either aerobic or anaerobic energy production depending on the intensity of the work. During exercise, the body makes use of anaerobic energy production because the body would not be able to produce the required amount of oxygen needed for the breakdown of Adenosine Triphosphate to produce energy needed by the muscles for contraction and expansion during exercise. But during slight activities that are not too vigorous, the body can make use of aerobic energy production because the body can cope with the amount of oxygen needed for breaking down the Adenosine Triphosphate to produce energy.

The food we eat is what provides our body with the energy needed for the workout. The workout can be really strenuous and requires lots of energy. It is very important to eat the proper food that would provide the body with the nutrients it requires for proper development. Our body gets nutrients from food in form of calories. Now we know that we have six (6) major classes of food but out of these six (6) classes, only three (3) produces calories for the body. They include the carbohydrates, protein, and fat and they are regarded as macronutrient because they are needed by the body in large quantities.

I have seen many people work so hard to build their body mass, they spend so much time, energy, and resources just to increase their body mass. But at the end of it all, they pay very little attention to nutrition, and I wonder why these people sabotage their success this way. If only they would just pay little attention to nutrition, they would be amazed at how much success they could achieve in a very short time. Most people complain that nutrition is very complicated, and they shy away from it. But the truth is that nutrition is not as complicated as people claim. Actually, if they can understand how nutrition works, then they would know how important it is and would utilize it for optimum development.

When we talking about nutrients for muscle building the first nutrient that comes to mind are protein, but that should not be so, carbohydrates are also essential. Carbohydrates are taken to supply body with energy. They can be found in foods like pasta, grains, fruits and vegetables, whole wheat bread and so on. But not all carbohydrates food supply the same quantity of carbohydrates to the body, some carbohydrates food supply more carbohydrates than others. Although carbohydrates are mostly given red flags in the diet world, carbohydrates still remaining one of the major sources that supply our diet with the most calories. It supplies our body with about 45-60% of the calories we need for our daily activities. While working out, it is very important to have a diet that provides you with the right amount of energy you need so as to gain the ultimate strength. If you follow the typical 2000 calories diet, this should mean that 900-1300 calories of your diet should be made of carbohydrates. Our body breaks down carbohydrates to produce glucose which is the body main source of energy. The glucose is a form of energy that can be used directly by the body when needed or stored and used when needed.

Our muscles are made up of proteins and water, to add a significant amount of muscle mass, a significant amount of protein needs to be consumed. Not consuming enough protein can leave some muscles lean and begging for attention. Proteins are also made up of amino acid which is important for cellular function and muscular repairs. Amino acids need to be available for muscle metabolism to release energy that is needed by the muscles. For example, to move any part of our body, we do that by contraction or expansion of muscles, for muscles to contract or expand energy must be present because energy is needed. Amino acid present in protein is also important for muscles anabolism (muscles build-up). The amino acids are broken down and stored in the muscles. Accumulation of this stored product is what results in muscle building. Just like carbohydrates, not all proteins are created equal. Some protein is more useful to the body than others; some are even more harmful than useful. When choosing the protein to consume especially when you are concerned with muscle building then you should go for proteins like lean beef, skinless chicken, eggs, whey protein and some others. Also in a basic diet of about 2000 calories, the protein should make about 10-35% of the diet that means 200-700 calories made of protein foods. Protein consumption could be higher for people who are concerned about adding muscle mass.

Fats are also one of the three basic nutrients that are needed by the body in large quantity. Fat can produce up to nine (9) calories per each gram of fat. Although some fats are unhealthy, the idea is to choose wisely and healthy. Fats can be really taken advantage of when considering adding muscle mass, but again the key is to choose healthy fats to consume like avocados, fish, olive oil, and others. Not eating enough healthy fat that can boost your body metabolism and regulate hormones can rob you from achieving ultimate body muscle building. It can also hinder the body from achieving its peak performance and diminish the body's function to build body mass. There's a popular saying "eating fat makes you fat", so get those healthy fats in your body and continue with your regular workout to develop those muscles and achieve ultimate strength. Also, in a basic diet of 2000 calorie, it is expected that the fat that should be present should be ranging between 20-35%, that is indirectly about 400-700 calories should be coming from fat.

You can also consider adding energy drinks and energy bars to your consumption. This is because most energy drinks and energy bars contains electrolytes usually potassium, sodium and chloride. Energy drinks and bar also contains sugar and a couple of calories. While working out, especially when working out vigorously, the body loses electrolytes through sweating. Consuming energy drinks and energy bars can help replenish those electrolytes really fast. Although drinking water is healthier. But during a vigorous workout, and the body has lost a lot of electrolytes, drinking water alone might not be enough to replenish the body of the lost electrolytes, so energy can come in handy at times like this. Moreover, most energy drinks and energy bars manufacturers add vitamin B to their products, as this can help be very helpful in helping the body metabolize energy-yielding nutrients (carbohydrates, protein and fats).

Chapter 2 (The Quality and Quantity of Nutrients)

What quantity of food am I to consume daily to achieve an ultimate body structure? Or what quality of food am I to consume? You may have been asked this questions a couple of times or better still you may have asked yourself these same questions. But the truth of the matter is that it all depends on what you are trying to achieve in your body. You may be seeking to add an enormous amount of body mass, or you are simply just seeking to lose weight and look the best. Now, these questions are twofold, first the quantity needed, and second, the quality needed. When the topic of weight is spoken of, most people focus is on losing weight. But to some people gaining weight is the goal. But gaining weight is not an open invitation to an eat-all-you-can buffet or an excuse to eat as much food that you can get your hands on. But whatever the case may be, a proper diet is what would enable you to achieve your desired goal. If you want a good result, you need to make smart decisions on what to eat, and a balanced diet is important. A balanced diet must contain all the essential nutrients, and most especially the macronutrient that is the carbohydrates, protein, and fat.

Normally, our body requires about 2000 calories to perform normal activities, but if you are seeking to add more weight then you would have to eat more calories than you consume. If you are seeking to gain weight slowly then consume additional 300-500 calories to your basic diet. But if you are seeking to gain weight fast then you should consider adding up to 700-1000 calories to your diet. While working out the body burns calories faster because working out requires energy. So if you just want to stay fit while working out, then consider adding 300-500 to a basic diet of 2000 calories so as to replenish the calories that were burned during the workout. But for those who want to add a considerable amount of body mass, then you should really consider adding the 700-1000 calories to a diet of 2000 calories. Our body can add about one (1) pound of body mass every week for every extra 500 calories consumed daily. Knowing that you need extra calories when working out is not enough knowledge to ensure your success in achieving your goals for working out in the beginning. You would also need to know more about the amount of calories that should belong to a certain food class, out of the number of calories consumed.

Consider carbohydrates, they are usually the highest in terms of quantity that are usually consumed in our diets. It should be ranging between 45-60% of our diets. That means whatever meal we eat should contain 45-60% carbohydrates. Our body can digest or absorb a maximum of about 60-80 grams of carbohydrates per hour during the workout. Technically speaking, the amount of carbohydrates your body needs depends on the type of exercise you are doing. Some workouts are more intense than others thereby requiring more carbohydrates than others. If you are into a normal workout routine of about 5-7 hours a week you should consider consuming 4-6 grams per kilogram of body weight every day. But if you are into a more intense workout routine that involves build building, and you workout for about 3-5 hours per day with 1 or 2 sessions daily, and you do this about 5-6 times weekly, then you should consider consuming about 8-10 gram per kilogram of body weight of carbohydrates spread throughout all your meal.

What about the quality of carbohydrates that needs to consume? Carbohydrates can be divided into 3 main groups; the starch, sugar, and cellulose. Cellulose cannot be digested by humans. Cellulase is an enzyme that is needed to break down cellulose but it is not present in the human body. The main source of sugar in our diet is glucose, fructose, sucrose, maltose, and lactose. There are also artificial sweeteners that do not provide any health benefits such as saccharine; there has also been controversy about its health safety. Starch is the main form of carbohydrates in our diet. Starchy food includes cereals, some fruits and vegetables, whole grain, nuts, potatoes and so on. When working out your body would require a lot of carbohydrates and you can get them from the food youngest. For example food like corn flour supplies about 87% carbohydrate, wheat supplies about 75% carbohydrate in general cereals should be a great part of your consumption.

Protein should not be left out of the picture because the body uses protein to build up lean muscle mass. So if you want to put on a decent body mass, you need to consider adding more protein to that diet. Some excellent food with dense calories rich in protein are the nuts like Peanuts, walnuts, almond nut, also meats are an excellent source of protein like beef, chicken, pork, even eggs are also excellent too. The quantity of protein to consumed should be considered especially when you workout and hoping to see positive results in a short time. For a bodybuilder hoping to add muscle mass should consume up to 2-3 grams per kilogram of body weight, which is equivalent to 400-500grams of protein daily. Even more, could be required depending on the vigorousness of the workout. But about 1.3-1.8 grams per kilogram of body weight of the protein can be consumed by people who are training just to stay healthy and in shape. You may be wondering as a builder training to build your body mass, isn't consuming so much protein bad for your liver, well it isn't. .

Quality of the protein you consume matters greatly. Not all proteinous food contains the same amount of protein. So when picking the quality of protein there are some major factors that should be considered. Firstly, you should consider that not all proteins digest at the same speed. Also, you should consider that some protein is better utilized in the body than other. Lastly, you need to consider the number of useful essential amino acids that the protein products can deliver to the body. Some people also supplement their diet with weight gaining protein shakes. Protein is excellent especially for those who are involved in a vigorous workout like weight lifting; the protein would help them to repair broken tissues and build the muscle mass. For example, beef when consumed and is digested, about 70-80% of the beef is used by the body. It also has lots of essential proteins that the body can utilize. Also, whey protein also digests really fast and about 90% of it is used by the body. It also contains essential proteins needed by the body especially leucine. Eggs too are also excellent but they digest slower than both beef and whey protein. About 90% of the egg consumed is utilized by the body. Eggs also contain essential proteins needed by the body.

Fat is also important because it can also supply the body with energy. You should have about 20-35% of fat in your diet, which is about 44-77 grams of fat daily if you are consuming the basic 2000 calories daily. Fats can be grouped into two groups; mainly the saturated and unsaturated fatty foods. Saturated fatty foods are not as healthy as unsaturated fatty foods. Actually, saturated fatty foods are one of the major causes of heart diseases, as it can cause high blood cholesterol levels. Eating healthy fat helps hormones function properly, especially testosterone for muscle development. Also, some essential vitamins that are fat soluble such as vitamin A, vitamin D, vitamin E, and vitamin K are also made available when fat-rich foods are consumed. Fat is also responsible for supplying the body with about 70% of the energy at rest.

The quality of the fat being consumed is also important. Some food products contain more fat than others. Keeping this in check is ideal. It is recommended to eat some type of fat because of their health benefits, and it is also advised to eat less of some type of fat because of their negative impact on our health. For example, unsaturated fat is divided into two, monounsaturated fat, and polyunsaturated fat. Not more than 15-20% of monounsaturated fat should be consumed daily, also not more than 5-10% of polyunsaturated fat should be consumed daily. Less than 10% of saturated fat should be consumed daily, and less than 300mg of cholesterol should be in our daily diet.

Chapter 3 (Nutrients Timing)

For those people who are into some type of workout or the other, whatever the reason may be, be it just to keep in shape, or to build muscle mass, or to lose weight, time to eat what to eat is a big game changer. When you do not eat what you are supposed to eat at the required time, you might not get the desired results you may be seeking. What to eat before and after a workout is a very popular question that has been asked numerous times by many people. To achieve that ultimate body structure you so much desire, it requires lots of effort and going through some major discomfort. Even with this, there are still some certain things that need to be in place. Some bodybuilding specialist would place you on a strict post-workout protein shake, while others just train you and tell you to eat what you can, the truth to achieving that ultimate strength lies in-between both spectrum. Slamming your body with so much protein shakes would help with weight gain, but might come with little or no extra desired effect on your body, in terms of gaining that ultimate strength. Also, you may decide to gain weight through a more relaxed way, but working out without a set of workout plan and timing those macronutrient targets, it may be harder and take a longer time to achieve the desired end you want.

You have your workout sneaker on, all dressed up and ready for the workout, but one thing is lacking which is food, yes food. What you eat before your workout, that is pre-workout is very important. Even what you eat post workout that is after workout is also very important. What you eat after a hard day workout is important because it helps the body recover from exertion; it also helps in building bigger and stronger muscle. Being thoughtful about what you eat before and after a workout is very important. I am not talking about workout supplements but really enjoyable food. Eating the right food can help energize your body for the exercise you are about to do.

It is important you know that for an effective diet, for those that are working out, it has to contain quality carbohydrates, lean protein, essential heart-healthy fats and fluids. Yes, fluids are also very important because while working out the body gets dehydrated. This fluid helps the body to stay hydrated and also to replenish lost electrolytes that could have been lost through sweating. Your muscles replies on carbohydrates like bread, fruits and vegetables, pasta for quick energy. Your muscles also require proteins like whey protein, lean beef, eggs, for repair of worn out tissues and to build muscle mass. Also, fats like avocado, white milk, fattier part of the meat, are needed by the muscles to provide energy to the muscles. There is no one meal to have for a workout but rather, consider having a low fat, moderate protein and carbohydrate, low fibre and do not leave out the fluid, it is very important. Having all these in your diet for a workout at the right time, then you are one step closer to achieving success in ultimate strength.

PRE-WORKOUT

Bodybuilder specialist always advises their trainees to always eat before a workout, as it would give them a better chance of getting the most out of the workout session. Not eating before workout can leave you feeling lightheaded, nauseous, and even dizzy too. This is because the body has depleted the energy it has in reserve and the body starts to shut down. Certainly, body part failure would be experienced too at extreme cases. Not eating can increase the chances of you getting injured, and if you do not get injured then you greatly expose yourself to negative impacts on your overall performance and always face reducing your gain.

Carbohydrates are one major nutrient that should be consumed before a workout. While working out the body uses glycogen which is stored in the body. If carbohydrates are not consumed before workout this glycogen gets exhausted and this leads to fatigue. The carbohydrate here should not be junk foods, but simple carbohydrates that can easily be absorbed by the body. It should be eaten 1-2 hours before a workout. Simple carbohydrates like fruits and vegetables can be consumed, or a special kind of sports drink can also be considered.

Protein is also very important before a workout. Any protein source can be eaten within some few hours say 1-2 hours before a workout, as this can help maintain and even increase muscle size. Mostly if you are into weight training, the process of lifting heavy weight could tear the muscles, protein are essential for repair of muscle damage, Also it can help lessen the amount of muscle damage, and make recover faster thereby improving your overall achievement.

Consuming fatty food also can be really helpful. When fatty foods are consumed before a workout, they can help to provide the body with essential fat-soluble vitamins the body needs. To top it all, fat can help slow down digestion, thereby keeping the blood glucose and insulin level balanced during a workout, making you stay on top of your game and keep you going.

You could also add a cup of caffeine to what you consume before a workout. It helps you stay alert and tireless, although the dose of caffeine is also key, an overdose of caffeine can make you feel nauseous and nervous. To top it all, in all these things you are suppose to consume before working, staying hydrated before a workout is very important. One way to check your hydration level is to check the colour of your urine before a workout. Just bit yellowish colour urine indicates proper hydration, but deep yellowish urine indicates dehydration.

DURING WORKOUT

While working out some certain things needs to be in place. More importantly, keeping hydrated is very important during a workout. If you are just going for a few minutes or few hours mild workout, water could do the magic for you in keeping yourself hydrated. But if you are into a more intense bodybuilding workout for several hours, then water wouldn't be enough to keep you hydrated. It's advisable you go for an energy drink. Also for proper and ideal hydration about 7-10 ounces of fluid should be consumed every 10-20 minutes during the workout.

Apart from keeping your body hydrated during a workout, you should also consume carbohydrates during a workout for energy. About 30 grams of easy to digest carbohydrates should be consumed every 30 minutes. This is because while working the body could get depleted of energy and this easy to digest carbohydrates would help replenish the body so that you can keep working out. You could consume gels, energy bars and so on.

POST WORKOUT

After workout out, it is normal to generally feel exhausted and weak. But eating after a workout helps to repair broken muscles and refuel the body of its lost energy. If you are unable to eat a full meal after a workout you could also have a snack then eat a proper meal a few hours later. But you should always ensure you eat after a workout. If you do not eat after workout then you would end up battling with low blood sugar and fatigue. You also face not achieving as much as you should if you do not eat, so it's best to eat even if you eat as much as just a snack. So we should endeavour to eat as soon as we can, especially after a really hard workout.

We need to also refuel our body with carbohydrates and proteins. Because we have used up a lot of the glycogen in our body and tore a lot of muscles, so we need to load our diets with complex carbohydrates to replenish the used up glycogen.

Also, we need to eat lots of healthy protein to repair the torn muscles. We need to eat a lot of carbohydrate or proteins, and we eat enough of it. Carbohydrates such as brown rice, nuts, whole wheat bread, and proteins like meat, beans whey proteins can be really helpful when consumed.

You also need to note that your protein consumption needs to be increased, especially for those that are into weight training. Apart from the turn muscles that needs repairs, we need to consume more protein to build muscle mass. Protein intake needs to be increased to 0.4-0.5 grams per kilogram of body weight.

Lastly, after a long tiring workout, it's important to rehydrate as soon as possible to replenish the fluids you lost while working out. Rehydrating yourself is even more important than eating. So endeavour to always rehydrate as so as possible after a workout.

Chapter 4 (Types of Nutrients to Avoid)

Working out to develop your body structure and looks takes time, dedication, persistence, and planning. You have to create time for it, fit it into your schedule no matter how busy you may be, push through, and be persistent despite how difficult it might be. It's a war you have to fight, and come out victorious. But with all the planning and persistence, and you eat the wrong food before or after or even during a workout session, there could be several complications. For example, you just step out of a treadmill and you are feeling really invisible and you think you deserve a medal for all the hard work, so you go for a block of extra cheesy cheese, but check yourself before you wreck yourself. After a hard workout, you need nutrients to replenish your energy and to repair your torn muscles, but some foods could just undo all the hard works you have been persistently pushing.

Meals that are hard to digest, filled with so much saturated fat or sugar, can do a lot of damage than good. Most especially when they are consumed post-workout when your body needs to repair itself. So with that in mind, we are aware that some food does more harm than good most especially for those hoping to train themselves for ultimate strength. You might not necessarily feel very hungry after a very hard work out, but it's advisable that you do not skip your post workout meals this is so essential because after working out you have depleted a lot of useful energy and your body needs to replenish this energy back and also repair itself. This is the really the ideal and best time to eat. It is really very important not to skip meals so that you can gain from every bit of the workout.

Having discussed so many healthy meals to have before, during, and after a workout, now let us talk about those foods that are not healthy for our workout development. Let us consider those foods we are to give a big distance to. The first foods on the list that we need to totally avoid are sugary foods especially during post workout. Why should you avoid sugary food especially after workout? Simple, it is because sugary foods slow down digestion. After a hard day workout, your body is depleted of nutrients and is crying for replenishment, having sugary foods would reduce digestion and delay the rate at which the body gets replenishment leaving the body starving. For example, protein smoothie is a really wonderful post workout meal because it helps to replenish the body and nourish it after an intense workout session. But you need to watch out because not all protein shake powders are the same, they vary. Some of them are heavy in sugar content or worse may contain artificial sweeteners. Simple, because they contain artificial sweeteners they could be harmful to our health. Majority of the artificial sweeteners are sweet to the tongue but bitter to our health. Moreover, these artificial sweeteners do not add anything substantial to the body especially after a workout rather it impends our progress.

Also, another food to avoid is the processed energy bar. This is a no-no especially for over processed energy bars with a long list of ingredients. Some energy bars are not bad for our muscles development, because some energy bar contains healthy sugar and proteins that can easily be assimilated by the body. Whereas, some energy bars do more harm than good. It's best to avoid energy bars that you are not familiar with all the ingredients. Most of the energy bars in the market are simply composed of sugar and they are no healthier than a candy bar. And I am not talking about natural health sugar, but refined white sugar that is high in fructose corn syrup with is very unhealthy especially for our blood sugar. If we seek to replenish our protein level after the workout we can do it naturally by consuming meat or eggs, and we can replenish out sugar level by consuming carbohydrates foods.

Low carbohydrates meals should be considered taken out of the list of what we consume. We may assume that carbohydrates are good and required by the body before, during and after a workout. In truth, yes they are essential for replenishing the glycogen that the body used during the workout, but not all carbohydrates meals are to be consumed especially after a workout. For example, low carbohydrates foods like; white bread, flour and even refined carbohydrates should be avoided. Rather, whole grain, fruits and vegetables can be consumed to replenish the body of what was used.

Avoiding salty processed food is also very important. After a workout, the body feels depleted of electrolytes through sweating, and it's only natural to have a craving for salty food, to replenish that potassium that was lost. But instead of going for those processed salty food, you could go for the natural alternative to replenish the lost potassium, with the like of banana. Even spicy food like hot pepper should be avoided because they are hard to digest and anything hard to digest should be avoided especially after a workout. Because the body is low on sugar, protein and carbohydrate, so easily digested food needs to be consumed at first after post workout so that energy can be restored.

One other food to avoid is fried food, health care professional's advice that we avoid this as much as we can. Fried foods were claimed to contain some types of fats that are not healthy, and they contain very little health benefits especially for deep fried products. Foods that are fried usually contain high-fat contents. High-fat content food should be avoided especially after a workout because they can slow down digestion and mostly after workout fast digestible foods can come in handy because the body is really depleted and needs to be replenished. It's also important to note that workout can be tedious and really stressful, so we also add to our diet, micronutrients and nourishing ingredients that fuels and take care of our body are needed.

High fibre foods and raw vegetables should also be avoided. Raw vegetables need to be avoided because after a long energy depleting workout, the body needs to recover, so at these times, really high-quality protein and carbohydrate are needed. But filling your stomach with raw vegetables wouldn't enable you to get the right amount of nutrients that are needed by the body. Also, high fibre foods need to be avoided especially salad and flax seeds. They may cause blotting. Instead, find what works best for you.

Among all these meals to avoid, the one we need to avoid the most is booze. If after a hard day workout, and you feel like just taking a break with a bottle of booze. Well, I am going to advise you to hold a full break right there, before accelerating into a sloppy curve down the overworking achievement. Booze is not the healthiest stuff to take especially after a workout. Booze dehydrates the body really fast and it also reduces protein synthesis.

Conclusion

Thank you again for downloading this book!

I hope this book was able to help you to understand the importance of nutrition, and know what you are expected to eat to get the most out of your workout session. This is so important because workout alone would not give you that desired look and goal you want except you combine it with healthy and effective nutrition.

The next step is to start figuring out those healthy diets that works best for you so you can achieve that ultimate strength and the sky would be your limit.

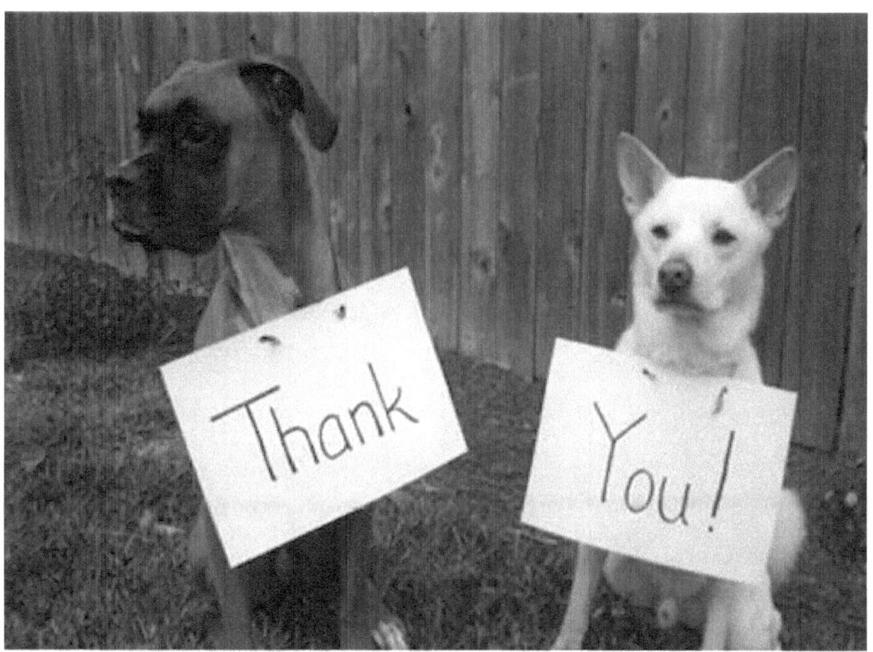

Finally, if you enjoyed this book, then I'd like to ask you for a favor, would you be kind enough to leave a review for this book on Amazon? It'd be greatly appreciated!

Thank you and good luck!

www.ingramcontent.com/pod-product-compliance
Lightning Source LLC
Chambersburg PA
CBHW051141250726
48655CB00007B/3179